RESISTANCE BAND WORKOUT FOR ELDERLY

BEGINNERS BASIC AND STRENGTH TRAINING EXERCISES FOR SENIORS

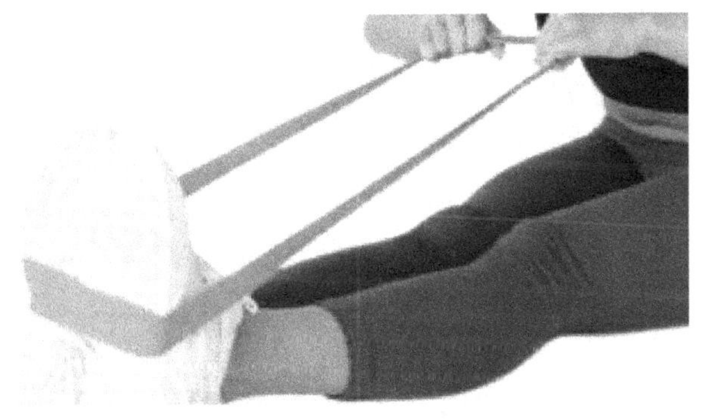

RICHARD E. MARSHALL

GET ACCESS TO MY MORE FITNESS BOOKS

INTRODUCTION

As we age, our bodies naturally change. We could lose flexibility, bone density, and muscular mass. Being active and carrying out daily duties may become challenging as a result. But as we age, there are many of things we can do to keep our vigor and independence. Training with resistance bands is an excellent method for achieving this.

Resistance bands are a versatile and affordable exercise tool that can be used by people of all ages and fitness levels. They are especially beneficial for older adults because they are low-impact and easy on the joints. Resistance band training can help to:

- Improve muscle strength and endurance
- Increase bone density
- Improve flexibility and range of motion
- Reduce the risk of falls and injuries
- Improve overall balance and coordination

In addition to these physical benefits, resistance band training can also have a positive impact on mental health and well-being. Exercise has been shown to reduce stress, anxiety, and depression. It can also improve cognitive function and mood.

Advantages for Seniors

Seniors who use resistance bands can benefit from a variety of health benefits, including improvements in their mental and emotional as well as physical health. Maintaining bone density, muscular mass, and joint flexibility becomes more and more important as we age. Resistance bands offer a low-impact way to accomplish these goals.

Strength and Tone of Muscles: By carefully engaging muscles, resistance bands enhance strength and tone of the muscles without putting undue strain on the joints. This is especially helpful for seniors who want to prevent their muscles from deteriorating with age.

Joint Flexibility: Resistance bands' elastic composition permits a wide range of motion, which enhances joint flexibility and lowers the possibility of stiffness. Maintaining freedom and movement throughout daily tasks is essential.

Balance and Stability: Improving balance and core strength, many resistance band workouts call for stability. An important aspect in reducing falls, which are a major worry for the elderly population, is improved stability.

Versatility and Accessibility: Resistance bands are readily available and adaptable, making them suitable for a variety of exercise regimens whether used at home or at a gym.

This accessibility encourages consistency, which is essential for fitness attempts to be successful.

The Importance of Safe Exercise for Senior Citizens

When it comes to the health of older persons who are physically active, safety is crucial. We'll talk about the special concerns and safety measures elders should take before starting a resistance band training program in this section.

Consulting with Healthcare specialists: It is imperative that elders get advice from healthcare specialists prior to beginning any new fitness regimen. This guarantees that specific health issues and ailments are considered, enabling a customized and secure method of resistance band training.

Appropriate Warm-up and Cool-down Techniques: We'll look at efficient warm-up and cool-down exercises that help the body get ready for activity and recuperate. These exercises are essential for reducing the risk of injury and enhancing joint health in general.

progressive Progression: Seniors should adopt a progressive progression strategy, especially if they are unfamiliar with resistance band exercise. The danger of strain or damage is reduced by gradually increasing intensity after beginning with less resistance.

Mastery of Resistance Bands

It's essential to familiarize ourselves with the subtleties of these very straightforward but incredibly powerful exercise equipment as we dig deeper into the realm of resistance band training. Comprehending the many kinds of resistance bands, determining the appropriate resistance, and managing and maintaining them appropriately are essential elements that can greatly influence the effectiveness of your exercise regimen.

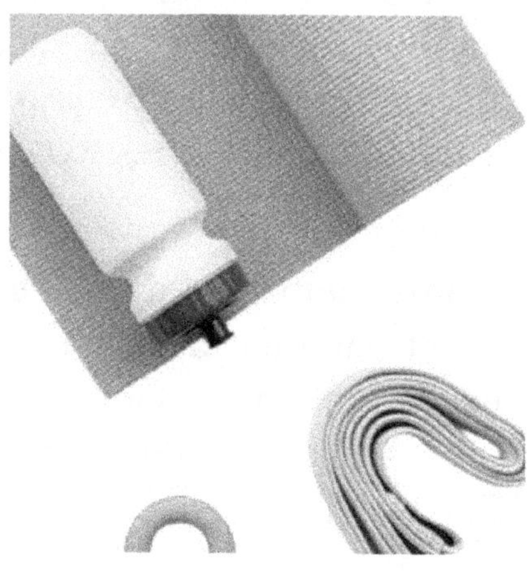

Different Resistance Band Types

Resistance bands are available in a variety of sizes and forms to meet different exercise requirements. Knowing the differences between these kinds will enable you to choose your workouts wisely.

Loop Bands: Leg presses and squats are two common lower body workouts that employ these closed-loop bands. They provide choices for users of varying strengths because they are available in a range of resistance levels.

Tube Bands with Handles: These bands are useful for exercises involving the upper and lower bodies and have handles on both ends. With their solid grip, the handles are perfect for exercises like leg lifts, shoulder presses, and bicep curls.

Figure 8 Bands: These bands, which have an eight-like appearance, offer two levels of resistance and are frequently utilized for workouts that work the arms, chest, and back. Their design presents a special difficulty.

Therapy Bands: Physical therapy and rehabilitation activities frequently involve the use of these broad, flat bands. They are frequently used in sitting or lying down postures and are great for mild resistance.

Knowing the distinctive qualities of every kind of resistance band enables you to customize your exercises to target particular muscle groups and fitness objectives.

Selecting the Right Resistance

A key component of a safe and efficient resistance band workout is choosing the right amount of resistance. Selecting the ideal level of resistance guarantees that your muscles are suitably strained or injured without putting you at danger.

Light Resistance: Light resistance bands are great for beginning strength-building and rehabilitation workouts, and they're especially great for newbies or anyone healing from injuries.

Medium Resistance: Those who have some workout experience and want to tone and strengthen their muscles should start at this level.

Heavy Resistance: Suitable only for individuals with a strong base of fitness, heavy resistance bands offer an intense exercise for advanced strength training.

It's critical to pay attention to your body's signals and begin with a resistance level that enables you to do exercises correctly. Higher resistance bands can be gradually added as your strength increases.

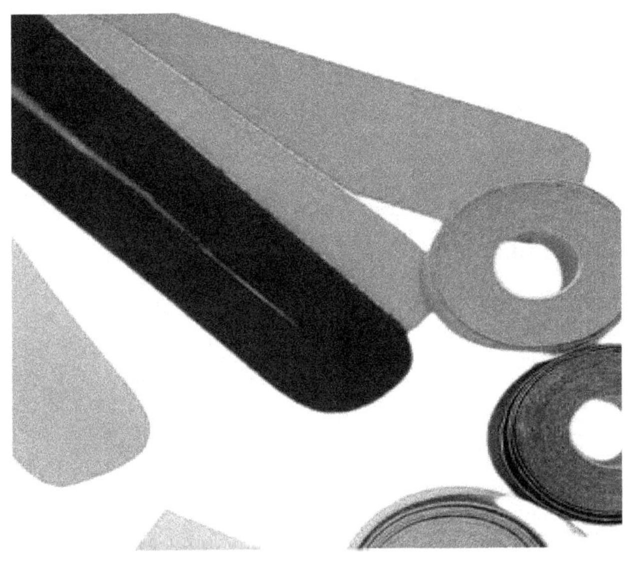

Appropriate Band Care and Handling

It's essential to handle and care for your resistance bands properly to extend their lifespan and guarantee a safe workout.

Examine Before Use: Check your resistance band for any indications of deterioration or wear before starting any exercise routine. If you notice any degradation in the bands, replace them to avoid breaks during workouts.

Safe Anchoring: Make sure your band is firmly attached to a sturdy surface before anchoring it. This keeps unplanned breaks from happening and makes working out safer.

Avoid Overstretching: Although resistance bands are meant to be stretched, going beyond what they can withstand might cause them to break. Make careful, regulated motions within the band's inherent stretch.

The right approach to store resistance bands is to keep them out of direct sunlight and in a cool, dry environment. By doing this, the material is kept from deteriorating over time.

CHAPTER 2

Basic Exercises for Seniors

With the bands, seniors can more safely determine how much they can push while lowering their risk of injury, making resistance workouts a valuable addition to any fitness regimen.

Here are a few general tips that apply to all of the exercises before we get into the particular ones:

- Don't overwork yourself and start off slowly. Recall that the goal of exercise is to promote long-term health. That doesn't include getting wounded.
- Start with a band that has a low resistance. There are several variations to choose from, so find one that you like. As you advance, you can always go on to more difficult ones.
- Always with your doctor before beginning a new fitness program. They can assist you in deciding what is best for your particular set of circumstances.

Seated Bicep Curls

Muscles Targeted: Biceps

Steps:

1. Take a comfortable seat on a chair and place your feet flat on the ground.
2. Ensure the resistance band is securely in place by placing it beneath both feet.
3. With your arms stretched all the way down, grasp the band's ends in each hand.
4. Curl your hands slowly toward your shoulders while keeping your upper arms still to work your biceps.
5. Carefully lower your hands back to the beginning position.

Reps: Start with 2 sets of 10 reps, gradually increasing as your strength improves.

Leg Press Variations

Muscles Targeted: Quadriceps, Hamstrings

Steps:

1. Take a seat on a chair with your feet flat on the ground and your back straight.
2. Using both hands, loop the resistance band around the balls of your feet.

3. Straighten your legs in front of you and push against the band's resistance.
4. Return to the starting position gradually while keeping your composure.

Reps: Begin with 2 sets of 12 reps, adjusting as needed based on comfort and strength.

Seated Row Techniques

Muscles Targeted: Upper Back, Rhomboids

Steps:

1. Sit on the floor with your legs extended, loop the resistance band around the soles of your feet.
2. Hold the ends of the band with both hands, arms extended in front of you.
3. Pull the band towards your chest, squeezing your shoulder blades together.
4. Slowly return to the starting position, maintaining controlled movements.

Reps: Start with 2 sets of 10 reps, gradually progressing as your back muscles strengthen.

Gentle Leg Lifts

Muscles Targeted: Quadriceps, Hip Flexors

Steps:

1. Sit on a chair with your back straight and a resistance band looped around your ankles.
2. Lift one leg straight out in front of you, engaging your quadriceps.
3. Hold for a moment before lowering your leg back to the ground.
4. Repeat with the other leg.

Reps: Aim for 2 sets of 12 reps per leg, adjusting based on your comfort level.

Chest Press for Upper Body Strength

Muscles Targeted: Chest, Triceps

Steps:

1. Place the resistance band behind your back at chest height as you sit or stand.
2. Take hold of the band's ends with each hand.
3. Extend your arms in front of you by pushing your hands forward.

4. Return to the starting position gradually while keeping your composure.

Reps: Begin with 2 sets of 10 reps, adjusting as needed.

Shoulder Press for Posture Improvement

Muscles Targeted: Shoulders, Triceps

Steps:

1. With the resistance band's ends at shoulder height, take a seat or stand on it.
2. Fully extend your arms by pressing your hands overhead.
3. Carefully lower your hands back to shoulder height.

Reps: Start with 2 sets of 12 reps, increasing gradually.

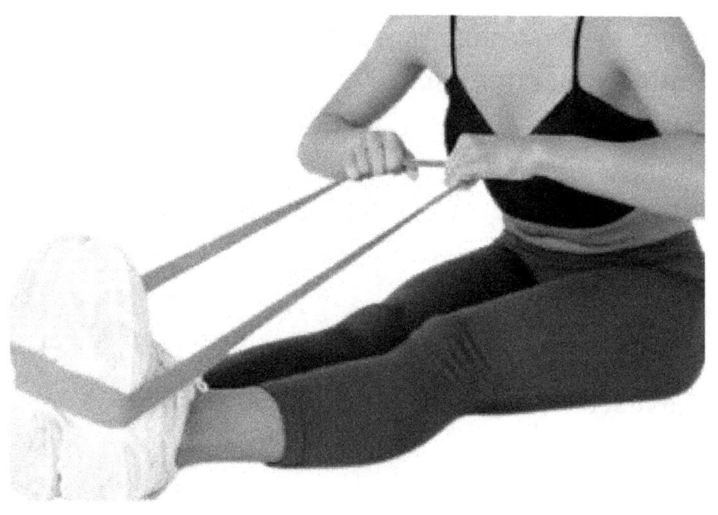

Ankle Circles for Joint Mobility

Muscles Targeted: Ankle Joints, Lower Leg Muscles

Steps:

1. Take a comfortable seat and hook one foot around the resistance band.
2. Raise your foot just a little off the ground and move your ankle in a circle.
3. To achieve a sufficient range of motion, rotate in both clockwise and counterclockwise directions.
4. Repeat with the other foot after switching.

Reps: Aim for 2 sets of 10 circles in each direction for each ankle.

Hip Abduction

Muscles Targeted: Hip Abductors, Outer Thigh Muscles

Steps:

1. Loop the resistance band around both ankles and take a seat on a chair.
2. To counteract the band's resistance, spread your legs apart.
3. Return to the starting position gradually while keeping your composure.

Reps: Begin with 2 sets of 12 reps, adjusting as needed.

Triceps Extension

Muscles Targeted: Triceps

Steps:

1. Take a seat or stand and place one hand behind your head to hold the resistance band.
2. Fully extend your arm and raise the band.
3. Return your hand to the starting position slowly.

Reps: Start with 2 sets of 10 reps per arm, gradually increasing.

Seated Leg Press

Muscles Targeted: Quadriceps, Hamstrings

Steps:

1. Loop the resistance band around one foot and take a seat on a chair.
2. Against opposition, extend your leg in front of you.
3. Using deliberate motions, bring your foot back to the beginning position.
4. Repeat with the other leg after switching.

Reps: Aim for 2 sets of 12 reps per leg.

Lat Pulldown

Muscles Targeted: Latissimus Dorsi, Upper Back

Steps:

1. Use a doorframe or other overhead support to secure the resistance band.
2. Take a seat or stand and hold the band with your arms outstretched.
3. To activate your Lat muscles, pull the band down toward your chest.

4. Take your time getting back to where you were.

Reps: Begin with 2 sets of 10 reps, adjusting based on your strength.

Seated Marching

Muscles Targeted: Core, Hip Flexors

Steps:

1. Sit on a chair with the resistance band looped around both feet.
2. Lift one knee toward your chest, against the resistance of the band.
3. Lower your foot back to the ground and repeat with the other leg.

Reps: Aim for 2 sets of 15 marches per leg.

Wrist Flexor and Extensor Stretch

Muscles Targeted: Wrist Flexors, Extensors

Steps:

1. Loop the resistance band around your fingers and sit
    or stand.
2. Holding the band at chest height, extend your arm in
    front of you.
3. For a little stretch, flex and extend your wrist against
    the resistance.

Reps: Perform 2 sets of 10 reps per hand.

Seated Torso Twist

Muscles Targeted: Obliques, Core

Steps:

1. Take a chair and encircle your midriff with the
    resistance band.
2. Maintain an extended arm position while holding the
    band with both hands.
3. Engage your obliques by twisting your body to one
    side.
4. Go back to the middle and do the same on the
    opposite side.

Reps: Begin with 2 sets of 12 twists per side.

CHAPTER 3

STRENGTH TRAINING WORKOUTS

Upper Body Exercises

Chest Press

Target Area: Chest, Shoulders, Triceps

Steps:

1. Maintain good posture while sitting or standing, making sure the resistance band is fastened around a sturdy anchor.
2. At chest height, grasp one end of the band in each hand.
3. Extend your arms fully and push both hands forward.
4. Take your time getting back to where you were.

Reps: 2 sets of 10-12 reps

Shoulder Raises

Target Area: Shoulders

Steps:

1. Place your feet shoulder-width apart in the center of the resistance band.
2. With your arms at your sides, grasp the band with both hands.
3. Raise your arms straight out to the sides while bending your elbows just a little bit.
4. Return your arms to the starting posture by lowering them.

Reps: 3 sets of 12-15 reps

Bicep Curls

Target Area: Biceps

Steps:

1. Place your feet hip-width apart and stand in the center of the resistance band.
2. Hold the band with your arms outstretched and your hands facing front.
3. Keep your elbows close to your torso as you curl your hands toward your shoulders.
4. Return your hands to the beginning position slowly.

Reps: 3 sets of 10-12 reps

Target Area: Triceps

Steps:

1. Place your right foot on one end of the resistance band.
2. With your right hand, hold the opposite end with your arm up.
3. Raise your arm and feel your triceps resist the movement.
4. Go back to the beginning and swap sides.

Reps: 2 sets of 12-15 reps per arm

Bent Over Rows

Target Area: Upper Back, Lats, Rhomboids

Steps:

1. Place your feet shoulder-width apart and stand on the band.
2. With both hands, grasp the band while bending at the hips and maintaining a straight back.
3. Squeeze your shoulder blades together as you pull the band toward your hips.
4. Lower the band back down gradually.

Reps: 3 sets of 10-12 reps

Front Raises

Target Area: Front Shoulders

Steps:

1. Stand on the band with feet hip-width apart.
2. Hold the band with both hands in front of your thighs.
3. Lift the band straight in front of you, shoulder height.
4. Lower the band back to the starting position.

Reps: 2 sets of 15 reps

Overhead Press

Target Area: Shoulders, Triceps

Steps:

1. Stand on the band with feet shoulder-width apart.
2. Hold the band with both hands at shoulder height.
3. Press the band overhead, fully extending your arms.
4. Lower the band back to shoulder height.

Reps: 3 sets of 10-12 reps

Target Area: Shoulders, Upper Back

Steps:

1. Place your feet hip-width apart and stand on the band.
2. Place both hands in front of your thighs and hold the band there.
3. Lift the band straight up, maintaining it in close proximity to your body, toward your chin.
4. Return the band to its initial position by lowering it.

Reps: 2 sets of 12-15 reps

Target Area: Triceps

Steps:

1. Stand on the band with feet hip-width apart.
2. Hold the band with both hands, arms bent at 90 degrees.

3. Extend your arms straight back, engaging your triceps.
4. Return to the starting position.

Reps: 3 sets of 15 reps

Leg Press

Target Area: Quadriceps, Hamstrings, Glutes

Steps:

1. Loop the resistance band around both feet and sit on a chair.
2. Straighten your legs and push against the band's resistance.
3. Take your time getting back to where you were.

Reps: 3 sets of 12-15 reps

Target Area: Quadriceps

Steps:

1. Sit on the edge of a chair with the resistance band looped around one foot.
2. Extend your leg straight in front of you against the resistance of the band.
3. Slowly lower your leg back down.

Reps: 2 sets of 15 reps per leg

Target Area: Hip Abductors

Steps:

1. Sit with the band looped around both legs, just above the knees.
2. Open your legs against the resistance of the band, then return to the starting position.

Reps: 3 sets of 15-20 reps

Target Area: Glutes, Hamstrings

Steps:

1. Place the band around your thighs while lying on your back.
2. Plant your feet on the ground and bend your knees.
3. Squeeze your glutes as you raise your hips toward the ceiling.
4. Drop your hips one more.

Reps: 3 sets of 15 reps

Lateral Leg Raises

Target Area: Outer Thighs, Hip Abductors

Steps:

1. At ankle height, fasten the band to a sturdy anchor.
2. Loop the band around your ankle while positioned sideways to the anchor.
3. Against the resistance, raise your leg sideways.
4. Return your leg to the ground.

Reps: 2 sets of 15 reps per leg

Hamstring Curls

Target Area: Hamstrings

Steps:

1. Fasten the band around a steady anchor that is close to the ground.
2. With the band looped over your ankles, lie on your stomach.
3. Bring your heels up to your glutes while bending your knees.
4. Extend your legs backwards.

Reps: 3 sets of 12-15 reps

Calf Raises

Target Area: Calves

Steps:

1. Stand on the band with feet hip-width apart.
2. Hold the band with both hands at shoulder height.
3. Lift onto your toes, engaging your calf muscles.
4. Lower your heels back down.

Reps: 2 sets of 20 reps

Target Area: Quadriceps, Hamstrings, Glutes

Steps:

1. Sit on a chair with the band looped around both feet.
2. Press your feet against the band, extending your legs.
3. Slowly return to the starting position.

Reps: 3 sets of 12-15 reps

Target Area: Quadriceps, Inner Thighs

Steps:

1. Place your feet together and stand on the band.
2. Move to the side while maintaining the band's tension.
3. Lower yourself into a lunge by bending the knee of the stepping leg.
4. Go back to the beginning and swap sides.

Reps: 2 sets of 12 reps per side

Core Strengthening Exercises

Seated Russian Twists

Target Area: Obliques

Steps:

1. Sit on the floor with your legs extended and the band wrapped around your feet.
2. Hold the band with both hands, lean back slightly, and twist your torso to one side.
3. Return to the center and twist to the other side.

Reps: 3 sets of 20 twists (10 each side)

Pallof Press

Target Area: Core (Abdominals)

Steps:

1. At chest height, fasten the resistance band to a sturdy anchor.
2. Hold the band with both hands at chest height while standing perpendicular to the anchor.
3. Hold the band in place for a little while pushing it out straight.
4. Put the band back on your torso.

Reps: 2 sets of 12-15 reps each side

Plank with Band Pull

Target Area: Core (Abdominals)

Steps:

1. Get into a plank position with the band around your wrists.
2. Pull one wrist up, bringing the band across your body.
3. Return to the plank position and switch sides.

Reps: 3 sets of 12-15 reps (alternating sides)

Bicycle Crunches with Band

Target Area: Abdominals, Obliques

Steps:

1. Lie on your back with the band around your feet.
2. Perform bicycle crunches, bringing opposite knee to elbow.
3. Pull the band with your hands towards the knee.

Reps: 3 sets of 20 reps (10 each side)

Target Area: Lower Back, Glutes

Steps:

1. Place the band around your ankles while lying on your stomach.
2. Using your lower back, raise your arms and legs off the floor.
3. Retrace your limb movements.

Reps: 2 sets of 15 reps

Target Area: Obliques, Abdominals

Steps:

1. Get into a side plank position with the band around your top hand.
2. Reach your top arm under your body and back up.
3. Return to the side plank position.

Reps: 2 sets of 12-15 reps per side

Target Area: Obliques

Steps:

1. Take a seat on the ground, stretch your legs, and encircle your feet with the band.
2. Twist your torso to either side while holding the band with both hands.
3. As you twist, keep the band near the ground.

Reps: 3 sets of 20 twists (10 each side)

CHAPTER 4

Cardiovascular Workouts

A comprehensive fitness program must include cardiovascular activity, especially for seniors who want to maintain or enhance their cardiovascular health. It focuses on designing customized cardio programs for seniors, utilizing resistance bands for low-impact aerobics activities, and the significance of heart rate and intensity monitoring for a safe and successful exercise experience.

Low-Impact Cardio with Resistance Bands

Benefits of Low-Impact Cardio, Seniors benefit greatly from low-impact cardio activities since they are easy on the joints. By providing an additional level of difficulty, resistance bands improve cardiovascular fitness and support joint health. Among the advantages include better heart health promotion, increased endurance, and improved circulation.

Examples of Low-Input Cardio Workouts:

- Marching as a group while wearing resistance bands

- Hold the ends of the resistance band in your hands and secure it beneath your feet.
- Alternately raise your knees to your chest while using your arms in a deliberate manner.
- Strive at a moderately fast speed while paying attention to your posture.

Reclining Leg Taps

- Place the resistance band around both of your legs and take a seat on a chair.
- Tapping your foot on the floor in front of you, raise one leg at a time.
- Maintain a consistent cadence while using your core to maintain stability and balance.

Adjacent Steps with a Band

- Encircle your ankles with the resistance band.
- While keeping the band taut, take side steps first to the right and then to the left.
- This workout strengthens the heart and works the hips and outer thighs.

Circles of Arms with Band

- Holding the ends in each hand, stand on the resistance band.
- Spread your arms out to the sides and move them in circles.
- This workout increases heart rate and works the upper body.

Marching While Standing and Reaching Up

- Grasp the resistance band firmly with both hands while standing on it.
- Lift your legs in turn, raising your arms above at the same time.
- This workout involves using both the upper and lower bodies.

Creating Senior Cardio Exercise Programs

Considerations for Developing Cardio exercises: It's essential to take into account each person's fitness level, medical issues, and preferences when creating cardio exercises for seniors. The idea is to develop engaging routines that get harder with time. As your fitness increases, start with shorter workouts and increase them in length over time.

Cardiovascular Low-Impact Circuit (15 Minutes)

- using resistance bands to march in place for three minutes
- Leg taps while seated (2 minutes)
- banded side steps for three minutes
- Band-wrapped arm circles for two minutes
- Five minutes of standing and reaching overhead

Tracking the intensity and heart rate

Heart Rate Monitoring: It is important for seniors to monitor their heart rate during cardiovascular activity to make sure it remains within a safe and useful range. Heart rate monitoring helps avoid overexertion and offers insightful information about the intensity of the activity.

Calculating the goal Heart Rate: For seniors engaging in moderate-intensity exercise, the goal heart rate is usually between 50 and 70 percent of their maximal heart rate. Subtracting their age from 220 gives an easy method for estimating their maximal heart rate. For instance, a 70-year-old person's maximal heart rate is thought to be 150 beats per minute.

Seniors should be encouraged to rate their perceived exertion using the Borg Rating of Perceived Exertion (RPE) scale, which gauges how hard they believe their

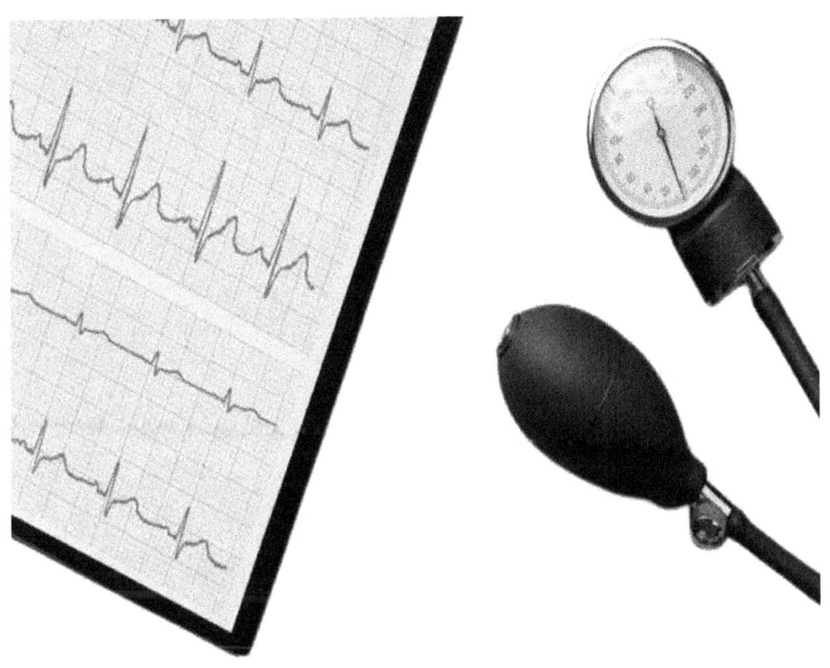

bodies are working. Aim for a moderate level that permits conversation while breathing is somewhat strained.

Using Heart Rate Monitors: Seniors can use fitness trackers or heart rate monitors for a more precise evaluation. With the real-time feedback these devices offer, users may modify their workout intensity to remain in the desired heart rate range. Stresses the value of adding aerobic exercise to a senior's fitness regimen and provides low-impact exercises using resistance bands.

CHAPTER 5

WEEK 1-2: FOUNDATION BUILDING

DAY 1: FULL BODY INTRODUCTION

Seated Bicep Curls: 2 sets of 12 reps

Leg Press with Bands: 2 sets of 10 reps per leg

Chest Press for Upper Body Strength: 2 sets of 12 reps

Ankle Circles for Joint Mobility: 1 set of 15 circles per ankle

DAY 2: CORE AND BALANCE

Seated Marching: 2 sets of 15 reps per leg

Standing Balance Rows: 2 sets of 12 reps per arm

Plank with Band Pull-Aparts: 1 set of 30 seconds

Dynamic Hamstring Stretch: 1 set of 10 reps per leg

DAY 3: ACTIVE RECOVERY OR LIGHT CARDIO

DAY 4: LOWER BODY FOCUS

Gentle Leg Lifts: 2 sets of 15 reps per leg

Leg Abduction with Bands: 2 sets of 12 reps per leg

Standing Balance Leg Curls: 2 sets of 10 reps per leg

Lateral Leg Stretch: 1 set of 10 reps per leg

DAY 5: UPPER BODY STRENGTHENING

Seated Row Techniques: 2 sets of 12 reps

Shoulder Press for Posture Improvement: 2 sets of 10 reps

Standing Chest Flyes: 2 sets of 12 reps

Wrist Flexor and Extensor Stretch: 1 set of 15 reps per arm

DAY 6-7: REST OR LIGHT ACTIVITY

WEEK 3-4: PROGRESSING THE BASICS

Continue with Days 1-5, gradually increasing resistance bands' tension and complexity.

DAY 6-7: ACTIVE RECOVERY OR LIGHT CARDIO

Intermediate 6-Week Program

Week 1-2: Building on Basics

Day 1: Comprehensive Strength

Seated Bicep Curls: 3 sets of 12 reps

Leg Press Variations: 3 sets of 12 reps per leg

Chest Press for Upper Body Strength: 3 sets of 15 reps

Ankle Circles for Joint Mobility: 2 sets of 20 circles per ankle

Day 2: Core and Stability

Seated Marching: 3 sets of 15 reps per leg

Balancing Rows: 3 sets of 15 reps per arm

Plank with Band Pull-Aparts: 2 sets of 45 seconds

Dynamic Hamstring Stretch: 2 sets of 12 reps per leg

Day 3: Active Recovery or Light Cardio

Day 4: Progressive Lower Body

Gentle Leg Lifts: 3 sets of 20 reps per leg

Leg Abduction with Bands: 3 sets of 15 reps per leg

Standing Balance Leg Curls: 3 sets of 12 reps per leg

Lateral Leg Stretch: 2 sets of 15 reps per leg

Day 5: Enhanced Upper Body

Seated Row Techniques: 3 sets of 15 reps

Shoulder Press for Posture Improvement: 3 sets of 12 reps

Standing Chest Flyes: 3 sets of 15 reps

Wrist Flexor and Extensor Stretch: 2 sets of 20 reps per arm

30 minutes of moderate-intensity cardio (e.g., brisk walking, cycling)

Week 3-4: Progressive Intensity

Continue with Days 1-6, gradually increasing resistance bands' tension and complexity.

Day 7: Active Recovery or Light Cardio

Week 5-6: Refining Technique and Intensity

Continue with Days 1-6, emphasizing controlled movements and increasing resistance for continued challenge.

Day 7: Active Recovery or Light Cardio

Advanced 8-Week Program

Week 1-2: Mastery of Fundamentals

Day 1: Advanced Full Body

Seated Bicep Curls: 4 sets of 15 reps

Leg Press Variations: 4 sets of 15 reps per leg

Chest Press for Upper Body Strength: 4 sets of 18 reps

Ankle Circles for Joint Mobility: 3 sets of 25 circles per ankle

Day 2: Advanced Core and Stability

Seated Marching: 4 sets of 20 reps per leg

Balancing Rows: 4 sets of 18 reps per arm

Plank with Band Pull-Apart: 3 sets of 1 minute

Dynamic Hamstring Stretch: 3 sets of 15 reps per leg

Day 3: Active Recovery or Light Cardio

Day 4: Advanced Lower Body Sculpting

Gentle Leg Lifts: 4 sets of 25 reps per leg

Leg Abduction with Bands: 4 sets of 20 reps per leg

Standing Balance Leg Curls: 4 sets of 15 reps per leg

Lateral Leg Stretch: 3 sets of 20 reps per leg

Seated Row Techniques: 4 sets of 20 reps

Shoulder Press for Posture Improvement: 4 sets of 15 reps

Standing Chest Flyes: 4 sets of 20 reps

Wrist Flexor and Extensor Stretch: 3 sets of 25 reps per arm

45 minutes of high-intensity interval training (HIIT) incorporating resistance band exercises

Week 3-4: Progressive Complexity

Continue with Days 1-6, introducing advanced variations and challenging tempos for increased difficulty.

Day 7: Active Recovery or Light Cardio

Week 5-8: Peak Performance

Continue with Days 1-6, emphasizing peak intensity and fine-tuning form.

Day 7: Active Recovery or Light Cardio

CHAPTER 6

When it comes to senior fitness, the idea of "no pain, no gain" is frequently replaced with a more sophisticated comprehension of "smart progress." Building strength while reducing the danger of overexertion or injury requires gradually raising the intensity of resistance band training.

Progressive Resistance: Choose a starting point for resistance that will enable you to do the suggested sets and repetitions with appropriate form. Gradually raise the resistance until the workouts become easy for you. This can be accomplished by varying the band's length or by utilizing bands with greater tension.

Incremental Reps and Sets: Make sure you can comfortably perform the prescribed amount of reps and sets at the beginning. Increase the amount of sets or repetitions gradually over time to keep your muscles challenged and encourage further progress. But always pay attention to your body, and don't push yourself too hard too soon.

Periodization: You might want to think about using periodization in your exercise regimen. This entails breaking up your training into several stages with differing degrees of difficulty. For instance, you may have two phases: one for developing endurance and the other for focusing on strength. Periodization keeps your training fresh and helps avoid plateaus.

Adding Variability to Exercise

Variety is the flavor of life, and resistance band exercises are no exception. Adding variety to your program guarantees a well-rounded approach to exercise in addition to keeping things interesting.

Exercise Rotation: To work on different muscle areas, switch up your routine by using different resistance band exercises. This maximizes the efficiency of your workouts by preventing the body from adjusting too rapidly. For example, rotate between workouts for your upper and lower bodies or between sitting and standing.

Testing Different Bands: Try resistance bands with various thicknesses and tensions. Different bands provide a more thorough exercise by engaging muscles in different ways. A variety of workouts may be made with a mix of figure 8 bands, loop bands, and tube bands with handles.

Including Functional Movements: To improve real-world tasks, incorporate functional movements into your daily routine. For instance, to increase general mobility and stability, simulate reaching, lifting, or walking. Including these exercises in your routines raises your degree of functional and useful fitness.

Tracking Development and Modifying Practices

Achieving greater fitness requires not just getting started but also keeping up with necessary adaptations. For long-term success, it is essential to regularly assess your progress and modify your habits.

Keeping a Workout journal: To keep track of your workouts, repetitions, and sets, keep a workout notebook. You may use this as a useful point of reference to see trends, monitor your development, and decide how to advance your workouts. Seeing your successes chronicled throughout time gives you a sense of accomplishment as well.

Listening to Your Body: Keep a close eye on how your body reacts to various workouts and resistance levels. You should adjust your routine or take a little break if you continue to feel uncomfortable or tired. Overtraining and possible injuries might result from ignoring warning indications.

Regular Assessments: Evaluate your general fitness on a regular basis, considering your strength, flexibility, and balance. Simple tests like gauging your reach, examining your one-leg balance, or assessing your capacity to carry out particular functional motions can be used to do this. Make use of these evaluations to pinpoint your areas of weakness so that you may adjust your exercise regimen.

Meeting with Experts: For regular evaluations and advice, think about meeting with a fitness expert or healthcare specialist. They may provide you feedback on how you're doing, make recommendations for changes, and make sure that your resistance band exercises are tailored to your particular health objectives and circumstances.

CHAPTER 7

Integrating Bands with Traditional Exercises

Enhancing Classics to Get the Most Impact:

Deadlifts in Opposition:

- Place a resistance band under your feet and use a deadlift grip on the grips.
- Constant tension is added by the band, highlighting the whole posterior chain.
- Keep your back firm and flat while contracting your hamstrings and glutes.
- Use bands to increase resistance during your deadlifts to improve your experience.

Band Walks Laterally:

- Just above the knees, wrap a resistance band over your thighs.
- As you walk lateral, keep the band taut at all times.
- By focusing on the hip abductors, this improves hip stability and avoids knee valgus.
- An easy-to-use yet powerful supplement to tone the hip muscles that are sometimes overlooked.

Triceps Reverse Kickbacks:

- In order to do a triceps kickback, anchor the resistance band and grasp the grips.
- Throughout the full range of motion, the triceps are challenged by the tension of the band.
- For best results, concentrate on a controlled extension and contraction.
- The constant tension of the resistance band will intensify your triceps training.

Defied Crunches on a Bicycle:

- Do bicycle crunches with your feet looped around a resistance band.
- In the crunch and leg extension stages, the band provides additional resistance.
- Benefit from constant tension while you work your obliques and core.
- With an extra challenge, turn a basic exercise into a dynamic one.

Band-equipped woodchoppers:

- Take hold of the handles with both hands and fasten a resistance band to a low anchor point.
- Cut wood in a diagonal motion, working your obliques and core.

- The rotating action is intensified by the resistance of the band, which improves core strength.
- Use the resistance band's dynamic pull to uplevel your woodchoppers.

Integrating Training for Balance and Stability with Bands

A Harmony of Power and Sensuality:

Ball Squats with Bands for Balance:

- Use a resistance band to enhance your squat technique while maintaining balance on a stability ball.
- While the band increases resistance, the unstable surface improves core engagement.
- This combination tests the strength of the lower body as well as general stability.
- Introduce the combined challenges of resistance and balance to up your squat game.

Banded Push-Ups using Stability Balls:

- While performing push-ups on a stability ball, wrap a resistance band around your back and hold onto it with both hands.

- The band creates unpredictability, necessitating more core involvement.
- Workes the shoulders, core, and chest all at once in a dynamic, hard way.
- Increase the difficulty of your push-ups by combining the band's resistance and the ball's instability.

Romanian Single-Leg Deadlift with Bands:

- Use a resistance band and do a Romanian deadlift while standing on one leg.
- The band engages the glutes and hamstrings by adding resistance during the hip hinge.
- concurrently challenges stability, balance, and unilateral strength.
- Increase the difficulty of your hamstring and glute workout by adopting a single-leg position.

Triceps Extensions in Balance:

- Using a resistance band, complete triceps extensions while standing on one leg.
- Engaging the core, the single-leg posture adds an element of instability.
- strengthens the triceps while improving stability and balance in general.
- Add the difficulty of balance to your triceps workout to make it more intense.

Band-Assisted Squats for Pistols:

- When performing pistol squats, loop a resistance band around a set point and grasp the other end.
- During the squat, the band helps with balance and control by offering support.
- tests the stability of one leg and uses the complete lower body.
- Increase the difficulty of your pistol squats by using the resistance band.

An Energetic Stretch Symphony

Shoulder Stretch using Resistance Bands:

- With both hands behind your back and your arms straight, hold a resistance band.
- Extend the chest and shoulders by gently lifting the band higher.
- The stretch is more effective as the band offers a regulated pull.
- Use the dynamic resistance band stretch to bring your shoulder flexibility program to a higher level.

Forward Bend with Bands when Seated:

- Sitting upright, wrap a resistance band over your feet and gradually pull them forward.
- The stretch along the hamstrings and lower back is made more intense by the added stress of the band.
- To increase flexibility and deepen the stretch, practice mindful breathing.
- Use the resistance band to increase the depth of your sitting forward bend.

Flex your quadriceps with band assistance:

- Place a resistance band around the ankle of the person standing on one leg.
- Pull the band gently to help stretch your quadriceps.
- The band offers a gradual pull that promotes flexibility and balance.
- Use the resistance band to help elevate your quadriceps stretch.

Dynamic Stretch for Hip Flexors:

- Place one knee on the floor and encircle the opposing leg's foot with a resistance band.
- Lunge energetically, letting the band intensify the hip flexor stretch.
- The resistance of the band gives the stretch a dynamic quality.

- Use the resistance band to intensify your hip flexor stretch and raise the bar.

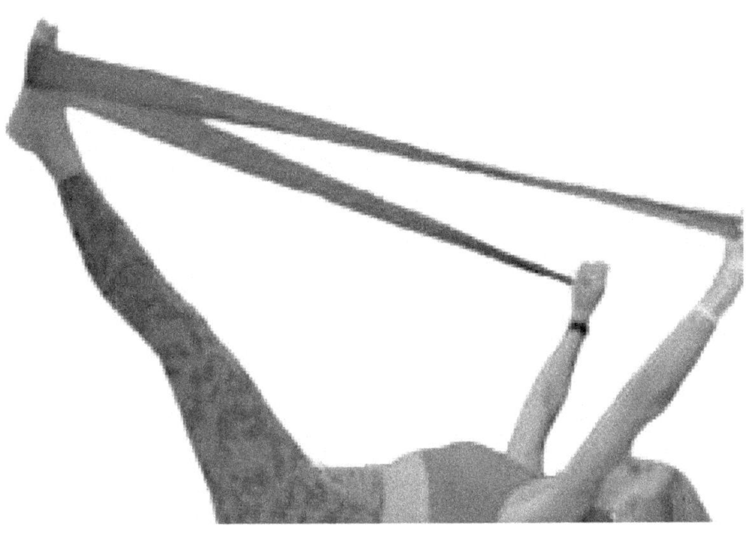

Flex your calf with bands:

- Place a resistance band around the balls of your feet while sitting with your legs outstretched.
- Feel the strain in your calves as you slowly pull the band in your direction.

- With the band's regulated pull, a deeper calf stretch
  is made possible.
- Introduce the dynamic resistance band aspect into
  your calf stretch practice to take it to the next level.

CHAPTER 8

Promoting Healthful Eating Practices to Support Fitness

Diet High in Protein: Seniors using resistance bands should place a high priority on eating a diet high in protein. For seniors to maintain and increase their strength, protein is necessary for muscle development and repair. Include foods high in lean protein, such as fish, poultry, legumes, and dairy, in your regular meals.

Balanced Nutrient Intake: Make sure your food is well-balanced and rich in different nutrients, including fiber, vitamins, and minerals. All the elements required for general health and vigor may be found on a colorful plate that includes a variety of fruits, vegetables, healthy grains, and lean meats.

Calcium and vitamin D: Resistance band training can help maintain bone health, and strong bones are essential for elders. A healthy diet rich in calcium and vitamin D is necessary for strong bones. To promote bone health, include dairy products, leafy greens, and fortified foods in your diet.

Staying Hydrated for Peak Performance

Importance of Hydration: Seniors who exercise in any way, including resistance band training, must maintain adequate hydration. Sufficient hydration promotes general cardiovascular health, controls body temperature, and preserves joint function.

Guidelines for Water Intake: Although individual requirements may differ, try to consume eight 8-ounce glasses of water or more each day. To avoid dehydration, seniors should be encouraged to consume water before to, during, and following resistance band workouts. Beverages high in electrolytes may be helpful, particularly after more strenuous exercise.

Keeping an eye on Hydration Levels: Elderly people should be alert for symptoms of dehydration, such as dark urine, lightheadedness, or lethargy. Sustaining ideal levels of hydration requires modifying fluid intake according to personal requirements and external circumstances.

What Are the Benefits of Resistance Band Training for Seniors?

Seniors who do resistance band exercise can reap several advantages, such as:

-Joint-Friendly Exercise: Low-impact exercises using resistance bands reduce joint stress.

-Variability: A variety of workouts for different muscle groups may be performed using bands.

-Enhanced Strength and Flexibility: Muscle strength and flexibility are improved with regular usage.

-Safe and Portable: Bands encourage consistency and are both portable and appropriate for usage at home.

How Do I Choose the Right Resistance Band?

Choosing a resistance band according to your level of fitness

Light Resistance: Perfect for individuals just starting out or concentrating on recovery.

Suitable for general strength training, medium resistance.

Heavy Resistance: Designed for more experienced users or those who want more intense use.

Can Resistance Bands Replace Traditional Weights?

Yes, resistance bands can effectively replace traditional weights, offering a safer and more joint-friendly alternative. Bands provide continuous tension throughout exercises, promoting muscle engagement.

Are Resistance Band Workouts Safe for Individuals with Joint Issues?

Yes, people with joint problems can safely engage in resistance band activities. Begin with minimal resistance and concentrate on deliberate motions. Before starting a new workout regimen, get advice from a healthcare provider.

How Often Should Seniors Engage in Resistance Band Workouts?

Seniors can benefit from resistance band workouts 2-3 times per week, allowing for adequate rest between sessions. Consistency is key, but always listen to your body and adjust the frequency based on individual needs.

Dealing with Band Snap Risk

Challenge:

Resistance bands may snap, posing a potential safety risk.

Solution:

- Regularly check bands for deterioration.

- Replace any damaged bands right away.

- Use the right methods to prevent overstretching.

Overcoming Grip Issues:

Challenge:

Maintaining a secure grip on the bands can be challenging, especially for those with grip strength concerns.

Solution:

- For a firmer grip, use handles or wrap the band around wrists.

- For improved traction, use bands with rough surfaces.

Adapting Exercises for Limited Mobility:

Challenge:

Some seniors may experience limited mobility, making certain exercises challenging.

Solution:

- Select workouts with sitting versions.

- Include assistive devices such as stability balls or chairs.

- Increase range of motion gradually over time.

Addressing Muscle Soreness:

Challenge:

Newcomers to resistance band training may experience muscle soreness.

Solution:

- Increase resistance gradually after starting with less.

- Include stretches for warm-up and cool-down.

- Drink plenty of water to promote muscle healing.

Seeking Professional Guidance

Challenge:

Seniors may be unsure about proper form or progression.

Solution:

- Consider working with a certified trainer experienced in senior fitness.

- Attend classes or workshops to learn correct techniques.

- Consult with healthcare professionals for personalized advice.

Balancing Safety and Progression

Challenge:

Finding the right balance between pushing boundaries and ensuring safety can be a concern.

Solution:

- Put form first rather than intensity.

- Increase resistance or the number of repetitions gradually.

- Evaluate your fitness on a regular basis and modify your training plan accordingly.

www.ingramcontent.com/pod-product-compliance
Lightning Source LLC
Chambersburg PA
CBHW070822280726
48660CB00017B/2601